Mohammed Maatallaoui is a Moroccan self-help writer who wrote the book *The Chemistry of Happiness Is Generated by Your Heart.*

He tries by writing this book to help people to live a happy life. By practicing the seven principles in this book, you can have the precious thing we call happiness.

Mohammed Maatallaoui

THE CHEMISTRY OF HAPPINESS IS GENERATED BY YOUR HEART

AUSTIN MACAULEY PUBLISHERS™

LONDON • CAMBRIDGE • NEW YORK • SHARJAH

A CIP catalogue record for this title is available from the British Library.

ISBN 9781398433045 (Paperback)
ISBN 9781398434660 (ePub e-book)

www.austinmacauley.com

First Published 2023
Austin Macauley Publishers Ltd®
1 Canada Square
Canary Wharf
London
E14 5AA

I would like to extend my thanks and appreciation to everyone who helped me write this book.

If this book has come to existence, it is thanks to the many people who helped me and gave me so many sacrifices.

Thank you all.

"Happiness has two principal basics: simplicity and kindness."

Confucius

Table of Contents

Introduction   11

Chapter One: There is no Hollywoodic Happiness.
     Forget That   16

Chapter Two: Even if You Are a Millionaire,
     You Need Work   29

Chapter Three: Don't Try to Be Successful and
     Powerful Just to Attract the Attention
     of Others   39

Chapter Four: You Are Already Rich   53

Chapter Five: Don't Resist Life Changes if You
     Want to Be Happy   65

Chapter Six: You Are Not Your Mind   83

Chapter Seven: At the End, You Will Die and
     (Me Too)…   99

Conclusion   111

Introduction

Perhaps the title of the book has come as a shock to you, dear reader. Because how can happiness be associated and attached to your heart? That seems strange and unusual. So how could that be?

Because most people don't live a happy life, as they are surrounded by the problems and conflicts of life from every direction and in different respects, the thing that makes happiness difficult for them and something rare to find it and achieve it.

So, happiness is a rare coin that is difficult to obtain in our life full of problems and difficulties. So, what can we do? And how can we achieve even a part of it?

I know that you want a clear answer to all these (previous) questions, dear reader.

Therefore, this book, which is in your hands now, will represent for you a clear map of the principles and actions that would enable you to possess that precious thing called happiness.

I know that talking about happiness in our world today has become something strange and unusual, as life has become a time journey full of pressures and problems, in which it is difficult for a simple person to follow the path of happiness or even to find it.

I know you might find this a little bit strange and suspicious too because many self-help books don't bring any real benefit to the readers. It may only represent a waste of money and time. Many of them are not useful. So how will this book bring happiness to you? I know that you would like to ask this question, dear reader.

Because most people assert that the person who is considered happy in our world today is just the person who became suddenly rich and has become a millionaire in one moment, and other than that is no more than empty talk. I know that you will have this thought as you read those previous lines.

Therefore, you expect me to prove to you the usefulness of this book, which is in your hands now, and to explain to you the benefit that you will get after reading it.

But my answer would be the opposite. I tell you, dear reader, about happiness of a different kind. It's different from everything you have seen in many Hollywood movies that represent the life of the rich and affluent people of America.

Most of what is promoted in these films is nothing more than Hollywood fantasies, which are inserted into the minds of viewers in order to establish a culture of consumption in various parts of the world, which is in the interest of major international companies and contributes to increasing their incomes.

However, unlike all the Hollywood fantasies promoted by those films, this book, which is in your hands, dear reader, will enable you through the actual application of the principles and ideas contained in it to obtain true happiness that stems from the depths of your heart.

This happiness differs from everything that is promoted in the audio-visual media and social networking sites.

Most of what they promote by these means is nothing more than a Hollywood illusion that is completely incompatible with the lived reality.

You, dear reader, cannot get the happiness that I told you about by owning a luxury car (for example).

You also, dear reader, cannot obtain it by adorning yourself with the most beautiful clothes of international brands and the best cosmetics (that's for women).

I am not talking to you, dear reader, about the momentary pleasures that these material things may give you.

No, because I mean something much more expensive than that, and a person can only know its value when he tastes it. I am talking to you about something that cannot be bought or sold, and you can never generate it with tangible material things. I am definitely talking about true happiness.

And in order to enable you to have it, dear reader, you will find this book consisting of seven parts, each part of which talks about one of the basic principles that lead by the practical application of it to the aforementioned true happiness.

Therefore, I hope that you, dear reader, will understand well these principles and begin after that to apply them effectively in your daily life.

You may find this somewhat difficult at the beginning, especially in our world today, where tangible material values have become prevalent.

This is because your value and happiness in this life have become measured based on the wealth that you own or the amount of money in your bank balance.

But I will assure you that every positive change is always punctuated by some difficulties and inconveniences that they are only in the beginning, which can be considered like a test of the sincerity of your intention. But they quickly disappear with time.

Therefore, I invite you, dear reader, to carefully read the principles and ideas contained in this book and to begin afterwards to apply them effectively in your daily life. The actual application is what will enable you to reach and enjoy true happiness.

This book is not that magic recipe that enables you overnight to enjoy the happy life you dream of. No, forget that. The magic recipe that can turn the scales is your usual actions and your daily lifestyle.

Therefore, if you want to live a happy life, the only thing that can enable you to do so is your usual actions and your daily lifestyle.

Hence, the goal behind this book is to help you live that healthy lifestyle which leads to that true happiness that I mentioned before.

Therefore, I wish you, dear reader, to read this book that is in your hands slowly so that you can benefit from it to the fullest extent possible.

I will now show you those seven parts contained in this book, which you will find as follows:

The seven parts of this book:

Part One: There is no Hollywoodic happiness. Forget that.

Part Two: Even if you are a millionaire, you need work.

Part Three: Don't try to be successful and powerful just to attract the attention of others.

Part Four: You are already rich.

Part Five: Don't resist life changes if you don't want be unhappy.

Part Six: You are not your mind.

Part Seven: At the end, you will die (and me too).

So, let's start, dear reader, by starting with the first part, which will discuss the validity and credibility of that Hollywood happiness that is being promoted through audio-visual media and social networking sites. Are you ready?

So let's get started.

Chapter One
There is no Hollywoodic
Happiness. Forget That

Every person dreams of living a life full of joys and delights in which he can realise himself and enjoy all its pleasures. I know that.

But is there, dear reader, an actual existence of this type of life? No, I don't think so. Not a single person in the history of humanity has lived this way of life. There is no such person.

Problems and trials are an integral part of this life. A life without problems and misfortunes is simply a life devoid of meaning and not even worth living.

What good is that you find yourself immersed in the pleasures and luxuries of life while at the same time suffering from a deep spiritual void and constantly feeling that your life is meaningless? The face of man to problems and obstacles is what gives meaning to his existence. In addition to that, that's also a measure of man's courage and the inner strength that he possesses.

Not only that but problems and calamities contribute to refining the human personality and also enable him to discover the hidden aspects of his being.

Thus, what many people may consider as curse can carry with it many hidden blessings that can help human to achieve and advance himself.

It is also not possible for a person to have a special identity or a high value in his society except when his life is associated with and contingent upon lofty ambitions and goals.

And when I say lofty ambitions and goals, I do not mean material things, a prestigious social position or even a certain authority a person has.

No, because all of that is doomed to perish with the passage of time, so none of that remains and lasts. So, when I say lofty ambitions and goals, I definitely mean those noble principles that a man possesses, which illuminate his life and give meaning to his existence.

As an example of this, we find success, helping others, honest and constructive work in all its forms and also many other noble principles that a person cannot offer anything positive to his society unless he possesses them. Otherwise, the person will be empty of identity and he cannot do anything good in his life.

Perhaps this can also be considered an explanation for why many rich people commit suicide despite the fact that they live in luxury and bliss. The reason, of course, is that they live without a lofty purpose, and they seek happiness through material things only.

The thing that leads them to increase their internal problems and exacerbate the spiritual void they feel, and unfortunately, this leads them in the end in a closed path in which they find no escape from depression and distress, and therefore, there is no salvation from that, except by suicide.

Life can never be sweet for a person who lives without lofty principles and morals. Because this is nothing but a path of madness and ignorance.

If we examine the biography of one of the great men in the history of all mankind, we will feel that he was living for a lofty goal and purpose, and he was not only living for luxury and momentary pleasure.

If Thomas Edison, for example, lived (only) for momentary pleasure, he would not have been able to invent the light bulb, which today is one of the foundations of modern technology.

Or if Steve Jobs (the founder of Apple) was also living without a lofty goal or purpose, he would not have been able to withstand the great problems he suffered in his childhood and youth, and we would not have witnessed the iPhone, which made a great leap in the world of mobile phones today.

Therefore, there is no escape from problems and trials in this life, as it is an integral part of it.

Every human being has a noble goal. He will necessarily be afflicted with various problems and calamities from which he cannot escape.

Therefore, he has only one of the two options.

The first is to confront it and seek only to solve it, which ultimately leads to that.

The second is manifested in escaping from it and trying to avoid it, which eventually leads to its aggravation and generates in the person many negative feelings about his situation, which may then make his life a journey of constant torment.

In fact, this may indicate that the person is devoid of principles, morals and values.

In order for you to understand this well, dear reader, I will tell you two true stories that confirm all this.

The first story is the story of Christina Onassis, the daughter of a billionaire and Greek businessman Aristotle Onassis, who was considered in his time as one of the richest men in the world, with his fortune, which was estimated to be about one billion dollars.

Christina was the legal heir to her father, Aristotle Onassis, after the death of her brother in a plane crash and her mother from an overdose of prescription drugs. Consequently, Christina inherited half of her father's fortune. Thus, she became the richest woman in the world in her time.

After that, she lived her life in luxury, as money was never a problem for her.

She owned many luxurious homes in various parts of the world, in addition to tobacco factories and import and export companies that she inherited from her father.

Consequently, Christina sought after that to live her life happily and enjoy her money to the fullest extent.

She had thought that she would get happiness from the outside world.

Thus, she decided to meet with her friends every day. She was left with no one else after losing her mother, father and brother.

Hence, she had hired them in her companies with huge salaries so that she could meet with them whenever she wanted.

She also married four times (with handsome men) but to no avail. All her marriages failed and ended in divorce despite the fact that she and her husbands enjoyed all the luxurious things in the world.

Christina Onassis owned the entire of Greek Island Scorpios (because it was part of what she inherited from her father), and she was constantly visiting the most beautiful resorts in the world of her time.

She had literally everything she wanted in this life.

However, despite all that, she was living in a long-term chronic depression that made her life a journey of misery and depression in stark contrast to the life of luxury that she enjoyed.

Christina struggled to live that Hollywood happiness that she was promoting through the American films at that time, but the result that she obtained was disappointing.

All Christina got was a life of bleak luxury.

Thus, after years of that dismal lifestyle she lived, Christina Onassis died at the age of 37, of a heart attack that many suspected was the result of her suicide by taking an overdose of drugs.

So this was the story of Christina Onassis, dear reader, who was considered the richest woman in the world in the eighties of the last century, and her life was a journey of depression and misery. Her grave mistake was that she lived a life without a lofty purpose.

A life based only on material wealth and deceptive outward appearances.

A beautiful life on the outside but empty and meaningless on the inside.

It's a really sad story; everyone thought that Christina was living a happy life full of joy.

But the truth was quite the opposite. Christina was living in a deep spiritual void that was getting worse day by day.

She really had a huge fortune, but she was missing much more important than that, which is the purpose and the reason of her existence in this life.

Christina did not have a mission in life, or even principles and values to live for. Her main concern in this life was just to harness all her material possibilities in order to live happily, which did not come to her and could never come to her in this way.

Rather, if this indicates anything, it indicates that Christina had grown up in an environment in which love for material things prevailed, but it lacked principles, morals and values.

Her life embodied proof of the impossibility of obtaining true happiness through money and material things only.

True happiness does not stem except from a healthy and pure heart filled with love for others and with morals and lofty principles, and whose owner has a lofty message in life.

Now that we have finished this story, I would like to ask you an important question, dear reader.

Still think you'll be happy only if you own a luxury car? Or that you only need a million dollars to be happy in your life?

I personally do not think so. Christina Onassis had all of that (and so much more).

But contrary to what you think, she lived a bleak and miserable life.

Even many doubt that this rich woman died by suicide.

So why, dear reader, do you live with these illusions and why do you curse your luck every day and wish you were born in a rich family and think that this is the only way to live happily?

While this represents nothing but an illusion in which you imprison yourself and torture yourself with it, the reality is completely different from all that. Money and happiness are different.

In my words, I am not calling you to live in poverty. Poverty is definitely not a good thing.

But I invite you not to delude yourself that money is what will bring you happiness. This is a big mistake, as money may cause you misery if you attach yourself and your life to it.

Money is just a paper. How can you link yourself and your value in this life to a bundle of papers?

You will live a bleak and miserable life if you do this, and you may eventually commit suicide.

Money role is giving you a life of luxury, but it cannot give you happiness.

Human happiness derives from his lofty principles and morals and also from his love to others and his good dealings with them.

If you want to live happily, dear reader, you must possess a noble message in life, which you derive from your healthy and pure heart that does not conflict with the principles and laws of life established by God.

In order to explain all this to you, I will tell you, dear reader, the second story, which is the story of a brown man from South Africa, considered by the whole world as one of the greatest men in human history.

He is certainly the famous South African man—Nelson Mandela.

Nelson Mandela was arrested in South Africa in 1962 arbitrarily and unjustly because of his demand for equality between black and white citizens and his rejection of racial discrimination in all its forms.

The authorities considered it an attempt to overthrow the regime, where racial discrimination prevailed in South Africa in that moment.

Thus, Mandela was sentenced to 27 years in prison, which he served in Robben Island and Bolsmore Prison, in addition to Victor Verster Prison.

But the strange thing about Mandela's story is that despite all the injustice and persecution that this great man was subjected to throughout that period of his imprisonment, his words always reflected the strength of his personality, his composure and his sincere love for all his countrymen.

The period of detention that this man suffered did not generate feelings of hatred and malice in his heart, and he did not consider it a disgrace to him. It represented to him clear evidence of his sincere love for all his countrymen and the sincerity of his case and his words as well.

He was offered several times his release in exchange for his cessation of demanding equality between all races. However, he refused this and preferred to remain a prisoner than to give up his case.

But after great international pressure for this, Mandela was released in 1990.

Three years later, that is, in 1993, Nelson Mandela was awarded the Nobel Peace Prize, which is considered global recognition and international recognition for this man for his courage, sincerity of his case and his words as well.

Therefore, this award was the conclusion of the life of a legendary man in every sense of the word. This man made achieving justice and equality among all races of the human race an obsession for himself and the source of his happiness as well.

He did not care about his opponents and enemies, and he never worried about them. They were too less to occupy the mind of Mandela. His main concern in this life was only to contribute to the achievement of justice and equality among all races of the human race.

Thus, he did not punish them after his release from prison (and after he was elected as the president of South Africa in 1994).

Rather, he forgave them all after they became humiliated and were under his authority.

His imprisonment for 27 years was a source of pride for him and a reason for his true happiness, which was always seen in his famous smile.

It was unlike Christina Onassis, whose life was a journey of melancholy and misery despite enjoying all forms of luxury, satisfying every whim and obtaining everything she wanted in this life.

Nelson Mandela was happy while he was a prisoner in that small cell whose area did not exceed six square meters (and under the most brutal conditions of detention).

The happiness of this man was not the result of material things. Rather, it was a real happiness that stemmed from his saturation with his cause and his words, his sincere love also for all his countrymen and his commitment to the noble principles and values that are represented in his struggle to achieve justice and equality among all people of different races.

So, this story is a clear proof, dear reader, that when a person lives for a noble and lofty goal and links his existence in this life to noble principles and morals, he will be entitled to that enjoyment of true happiness which his pure and healthy heart becomes a source for.

As a conclusion to this part, I would like you, dear reader, to search in yourself and your entity for the lofty principles and morals that you love and would like to live for, such as tolerance (for example), love of good for others, honourable work or unconditional giving...

After that, you begin to associate yourself and your existence in this life with those morals and principles.

By doing this, you will improve your feelings, feelings and psychological state in general, as it will gradually allow you to enjoy the true happiness that I told you about.

First Wisdom

True happiness is felt by a person who has lofty principles and morals and who also has a noble goal and a lofty mission in life to live for.

Material things cannot generate real and permanent happiness because their role is limited only to enabling human to live in luxury.

Chapter Two
Even if You Are a Millionaire, You Need Work

Yes, dear reader, even if you are rich and a millionaire, you are in dire need to work. Work is what gives you value in this life.

This may be shocking you. Everyone believes that if a person is rich, he will not need to work.

But this is nothing more than an illusion that prevails and is widespread in our time. Like it or not, we are in deep need to work.

Because if a person does not find a job for himself in his society, he will certainly become a corrupt person, which will lead him to destroy himself and waste his future as well.

When a person does not do something, he will gradually begin to deviate and go astray. And he will find himself (little by little) starting to do many negative and deviant actions, such as alcoholism or drug abuse (in all its forms).

And all of this is generated from one and only thing; it is the free time (certainly). The free time is fatal and destructive, dear reader. Therefore, even if a person is a millionaire, he is in dire need of work.

Work is the only positive thing in which a person can put his energy and occupy his time.

It is not by chance that we find that most of the people who are corrupt don't do their work as they should and also do many deviant acts such as drug abuse and alcoholism.

So whether we like it or not, work is an inseparable part of life; life cannot be good except by work. Work and work. Nothing can be better than work. Work is the best thing.

A person cannot live happily unless he performs a certain action and positively affects his society.

Rather, even if a person is a millionaire, he needs to do something in order to fill his life by happiness.

In order to explain this to you in a more realistic way, I will tell you, dear reader, the story of an English young man who was considered in 2002 as one of the richest people in the city of Swaffham (England), but he lived a miserable life and ended up in bankruptcy in the year 2012.

It is certainly the young Englishman Mike Carroll.

Mike Carroll won $12 million in a gambling contest in 2002. Thus, he became one of the rich people of his town (the town of Swaffham, which is located in the north of London).

He became very famous and became the focus of all people's attention. In fact, he appeared in many famous television programmes, such as the programme *Beer and Pizza* (which was a well-known programme at that time).

But this young Englishman (Mike Carroll) was not thinking like other rich people to invest his money in a project or even to do a specific job in his life.

He only wanted to hang out with his money and spend it in nightclubs and drug addiction (cocaine). But he did not know that he was leading his life into the abyss through those reckless and perverted acts and that negative lifestyle.

He was not doing any work. Thus, in addition to living a bleak life as a result of that bad lifestyle, he ended up (also) in bankruptcy in 2012.

After only ten years of extravagance, (Mike Carroll) spent everything he received in that prize ($12 million), and nothing was left of it.

Consequently, he was forced to leave his city and to settle in the Scottish city—Elgin, where he began to work as a woodcutter and charcoal seller for a wage of $12 an hour (only).

Carroll describes what happened to him by saying that what comes easily goes easily.

The money that a person obtains from gambling can only be spent on drugs, nightclubs and women (I mean prostitution).

And the story of this young Englishman is the best proof of that.

Mike Carroll continues his talk by saying that he is living a happier life now because he works every day and does something positive in his life.

So this sad story, dear reader, is considered the best evidence that when a person works and does something (a positive role in his society), it allows him to live happily.

Mike Carroll won more than $12 million in that prize (gambling), but he lived a bleak and miserable life and eventually went bankrupt.

Life, dear reader, can never be good until you do something and you positively affect your society.

I know, dear reader, that there is a major problem that most young people suffer from unemployment. That is, there are many young people who would like to work, but they cannot find jobs.

But I will tell you, dear reader, an important fact, which is that the main reason for the unemployment problem is not the lack of jobs but rather the lack of a qualified workforce.

As many of the young people who hold higher degrees are not qualified to work in the positions provided by the labour market. This is due to only two main factors: The first is manifested in the weakness of the educational system, and this problem is widespread and prevalent in most countries of the world, where education is no longer compatible with the requirements of the labour market.

To overcome this problem, there is only one solution, which is self-education.

That is, the student should not limit himself to what he learns at school or university but also teach himself.

A student can learn many different subjects through the internet or by reading books.

As for the second factor that makes the workforce unqualified, it is the weakness of the human factor.

That is, there are many young people today who are not interested in their future, and they only want to hang out and use drugs and also do many perverted acts which make them unable to do any work (and also make them suffer from unemployment).

I think that these two reasons that I mentioned to you, dear reader, explain the reason for the existence of the unemployment problem. A person who wants to work and be useful in his society (and to play a positive role in it) must get an opportunity to work.

Even if he suffers from unemployment for a certain period, he will eventually be able to enter the job market.

As for people (who do not want to work in a job) and want to establish their own business, this will not be easy (of course) at the beginning. But with some persistence, perseverance and patience over the travails of circumstances, the person will eventually be empowered to establish his own business or project.

As my advice to you, dear reader, in this context (of course if you want to establish your own business), it is important for you to choose the field in which you want to work.

Because if you want to work in a certain field only for money, you will not be able to continue until the end. You will also not be patient with the difficulties and problems that you will encounter in the beginning.

You will end up withdrawing and not wanting to continue. Therefore, it is important for you, dear reader, to work in the field that you love, and in which you feel that you have peace of mind while you work in it because this is one of the most important success keys.

In addition to that, it is important that you also know, dear reader, the secrets of the work you want to do.

In order to be able to do this, you have to look for people who do the same work (that you want to do). And try to take some valuable information and advice from them because this will help you a lot and will make it easier for you.

Also, it is not just about those things, but there is also the mental aspect. Because for the person who wants to establish his own business, it is also important for him to have a great mentality.

As an advice to you (from me) in this context, dear reader, I will direct you to a set of books that will help you acquire the mindset of an entrepreneur, and which also provide you with a set of valuable advice in the financial field—books: *Secrets of the Millionaire Mind*, *The Richest Man in Babylon*, *Rich Dad Poor Dad*, *The Secret*, *The Alchemist*, *Daily Teachings*, *The Hero* and *Who Moved My Cheese?*

As a summary of this part, I will assure you, dear reader, of an important fact.

That is, human happiness is closely related to work.

A person who does not play a positive role in his society can never be happy. Work is one of the most important factors generating human happiness.

I know that it will come to your mind, dear reader, that there are many people who work and play a positive role in their society, but despite all that, they live in constant and semi-permanent misery and suffering. Rather, their work may be the cause of their misery and pain. How is it possible for work to generate happiness and at the same time cause misery and pain for these good people?

The answer to your question, dear reader, is simple.

The problem that these people suffer from is not the work itself because work can never be a negative thing.

The problem with these people is that they work in fields they do not like (just for the money). After that, they find themselves stuck in that kind of life that they do not like, and life seems dark in their eyes.

And I will assure you, dear reader, that there is only one solution to this problem, and that is to start looking for the work they like to do. And try after that (albeit gradually) to change their job or their own work in which they work.

I know that this will be somewhat difficult at first, as there are a lot of expenses that we must pay (monthly).

But I will assure you, dear reader, that if you find sincere contentment and insistence on a certain thing, then it can definitely be achieved and reached.

This problem has faced many people (who are today successful, millionaires and happy as well) and they managed to overcome it.

So if you, dear reader, suffer from this, do not let your fear make you work in that work that you don't like and live in constant misery.

If you do not like your job, try to leave it as soon as possible. And start looking for a job that you love and you will like to do (even if it might be difficult at first).

And if you want to do your own business, then start now. I know it will be difficult at first. But you will overcome these difficulties if you believe in yourself; you can do that. Don't forget that God does not burden a soul beyond its capacity, and as long as He has put you in this situation in which you are currently, He has (also) appointed for you the appropriate solution for it.

So, dear reader, follow your intuition and your inner sense and start looking for the work you love and want to do. After you have overcome those obstacles and difficulties that you will suffer from in the beginning, you will find that they have made you a more powerful person, and soon you will discover that you are going in the right direction.

And that your own work (or your new job) has made of you another person, a happy and strong person full of joy, joy and optimism.

And when you become like that, you will flourish even in your business and you will succeed in it. Happiness leads to success as well.

So, dear reader, I advise you to work, work is one of the most important sources of happiness in the human life.

If you want happiness in your life, you must do the work that you love, which makes you a positive and beneficial person for himself and his society.

Whatever the person's financial condition is, he needs work to live a happy life.

Even if a person is a millionaire, he needs work.

Wisdom
Part Two

Work is an essential thing in the life of every human being, as it is one of the most important factors that generate happiness.

When a person does a job that he loves, he leads his life to prosperity in all aspects:

* The spiritual side
* The material side
* The emotional side

Chapter Three
Don't Try to Be Successful and Powerful Just to Attract the Attention of Others

In 1991, Pablo Escobar had a golden opportunity. The Colombian government offered him to spend only five years in La Catedral Prison as punishment for all his past actions and crimes, which is represented in drug trafficking (cocaine) and smuggling it to the United States of America in addition to killing hundreds of citizens in Colombia, even its former presidential candidate—Luis Carlos Galan.

Five years is nothing compared to the criminal record that Escobar possesses, as he is considered one of the most dangerous criminals in history.

Colombia lived one of its worst periods in the era of this criminal. (He was behind the killing of more than 2000 people in Colombia).

Pablo accepted the offer and moved to La Catedral Prison, the construction of which he personally supervised.

Thus, it was not similar to other prisons except in the name. It was a five-star hotel called a prison, where Pablo Escobar's cell was a large room equipped with imported furniture, and also had a large TV screen so that (Pablo) could watch his favourite movies, and a large bathroom to maintain his personal hygiene.

As for the rest of the prison facilities, it contained many entertainment facilities in addition to a nightclub for Pablo and his men to celebrate. There were also the finest wines and many beautiful women (the most beautiful women of Colombia) and even football fields and sports spaces.

La Catedral was in fact a five-star hotel, not a prison.

All that was required of Pablo was to abandon his criminal activities.

But he could not do that, as he did not fulfil his promise to the Colombian government. Soon he returned to drug dealing, as he was running his business from inside the prison.

Pablo was at the height of his power. Forbes magazine ranked him as the seventh richest man in the world in 1989, with his fortune estimated at about $30 billion. (Escobar was actually the seventh richest man in the world, as he made a huge fortune from that dirty work which he was doing).

But was money all that Pablo was looking for? The answer, of course, is no. Otherwise, he would not have broken his promise to the Colombian government.

So why then did Pablo Escobar return to drug dealing despite being extremely wealthy and having no need to do that dirty work?

The answer, dear reader, is simply that Escobar had become fond of imposing his power and influence on others (dominate them). He wanted to impress others and always look brave and strong.

He always wanted to be the centre of people's attention and the source of their admiration.

He did so in various ways, building homes for the poor in many slums in Colombia, and even hospitals and schools as well.

The apparent goal was for Pablo to provide humanitarian aid to the people of his town. But the hidden goal behind this was manifested in his desire to extend his power and influence in the Colombian city of Medellin, which we grew up in.

Pablo was really addicted to that because this was what fuelled his arrogance and greatness.

In order to be able to do so, he was in dire and constant need of money.

Money was the only thing that would allow him to do that.

Thus, Escobar began to think that the more money he had, the more he would be able to gain the respect and appreciation of others (but this was only an illusion in his mind).

Therefore, money was his only goal in this life, as he was insatiable with it. But he was getting thirsty for him day by day. It is the only thing that fuels his arrogance (and his megalomania too).

Thus, Escobar became addicted to getting more money.

This was the real reason why he was unable to fulfil his promise to the Colombian authorities.

Soon, Escobar returned to drug dealing from inside La Catedral Prison and further expanded his trade.

But he was not aware that the breach of his promise had missed a golden opportunity.

After the Colombian authorities know of this, they wanted to transfer him to a real prison in order to tighten the noose on him further. Pablo knows about this and did not find an alternative to escaping from prison, which increased the anger of the Colombian authorities on him. So, in agreement with the American forces, they launched a massive campaign against him in order to return him to prison or even extradite him to the United States of America, where the punishment would be more severe.

The extradition of criminals to the United States of America was Pablo Escobar's biggest fear, as he would have preferred to die in Colombia than to be a prisoner in the United States of America.

If he was extradited to the United States of America, the penalty there may reach life imprisonment.

Consequently, he found only one solution in front of him, which was to hide from the authorities and hide from view.

But that didn't work in the end. After a year of tracking, the Colombian police, with the help of US forces, were able to locate Escobar and end the long pursuit that lasted for a year and a half.

Thus, Escobar was killed in 1993 by the Colombian authorities. (NB: There are those who say that Escobar committed suicide after being besieged by Colombian forces).

This was the end of the story of this criminal, who can be considered one of the most dangerous criminals throughout history.

That was the story of Pablo Escobar, dear reader, that the dangerous criminal who killed more than 3000 Colombian citizens blew up many Colombian installations and also killed many innocent civilians. This criminal struck terror into the hearts of all Colombians, but his end was horrible.

Thus, the lesson can be taken from Escobar's story, as it embodies a living example that success, whose goal is only to draw the attention of others and gain their admiration, often has a tragic end.

Because when a person strives for only that, he will definitely take illegal ways in order to obtain that success as soon as possible.

This kind of success can never be achieved through legitimate means.

Because the success that is achieved by legitimate means often requires great time and effort in order to achieve it.

Thomas Edison, for example, could not invent the light bulb until after great time and effort. He tried about 10,000 attempts before he finally managed to invent it.

Therefore, the success whose purpose is only to impress others can never be achieved by legitimate means. Rather, it will always be either through drug trafficking, fraud or other illegal acts.

Therefore, I invite you, dear reader, not to seek success just to impress others because if you do that, you will inevitably strive to achieve that success in any way, and therefore you will choose the illegal ways because it is the only one that allows you to achieve this success quickly.

Success that is motivated only by drawing the attention of others can never be achieved by legitimate means.

Rather, it will always come through the commission of many vile acts and crimes, the consequences of which will be serious in the end.

Juan Pablo Escobar (son of Pablo Escobar) stated that his father was not living happily but was living in constant and permanent misery, where he was always wary of his enemies and the Colombian authorities as well, even from Colombia signing the extradition agreement to the United States of America, according to which it was able to extradite him (Pablo Escobar) to the United States of America, where he was to be imprisoned there for life as a punishment for all his terrible deeds and crimes that he had committed (which clearly indicates the extent of the suffering that he suffered).

The success that has the sole goal of impressing others can only be the result of deep internal problems that man suffers from, as he wants to escape through that success from his psychological complexes and deep internal conflicts in addition to the fact that he also wants to satisfy his ego and pride (through get-that kind of success).

However, he then finds himself addicted to achieving material success through illegal and immoral acts.

Escobar, for example, was in the year 1991 one of the richest men in the world with his huge fortune, which was estimated at about 30 billion dollars.

That is, he never needed the money. When a person has 30 billion dollars, he can provide for all his material needs, his children and his family (and his town as well).

Rather, this amount is considered the budget of many countries.

If Pablo does not need the money, then what is the motive that made him return to that dirty work (drug trafficking)?

The answer, of course, is that Escobar became addicted to getting (more) money illegally and even became thirstier to do so.

In addition, when a person gets involved in this dirty work, he can never get out of it because if he does that, his partners will kill him. That means the end is always imprisonment or death, as there is nothing else.

So I hope, dear reader, that you take the story of this criminal as an example. Indeed, the opposite of what is being promoted by some films and series that embody the story of

Pablo Escobar, where he is portrayed as a popular hero or (Robin Hood of Colombia) who steals from the rich of America and helps the poor of the Colombian city of Medellin.

The reality is contrary to all of this. All of this is nothing more than nonsense.

Pablo Escobar was responsible for the deaths of many civilians and poor people in Colombia. Or rather, more than 3,000 Colombian citizens, including civil servants and ordinary citizens in addition to policemen and soldiers.

Even young children who are not guilty, Escobar had killed them in the bombings he was carrying out in the city of Bogota (the capital of Colombia) in order to pressurise the Colombian authorities not to ratify the law on extradition to the United States of America.

In other words, all that Pablo Escobar was interested in was only the success of his trade which he was doing, which made him a criminal (and a killer as well) who killed anyone that disagreed with his opinion.

So I am very surprised when I see many people consider Pablo Escobar as a hero or as an inspiration to them.

Whereas, all that he mattered about was that he become richer (in any way). And all this to dominate others like he wants, in order to attract their attention and admiration for him (in order to feed his pride and arrogance through this).

So I hope, dear reader, that you benefit from the story of Escobar and his tragic end. And take this as evidence that success, whose aim is only to attract the attention of others and impress them, is always accompanied by misery and unhappiness and can never be achieved except through dirty and immoral (and also illegal) actions, which makes the end of its owner tragic.

I know that you, dear reader, would now like to know the other kind of success, which is obtained by legitimate means.

If the motive behind success in illegal ways is to draw the attention and admiration of others in order to satisfy vanity, pride and megalomania, what is the motive then to achieve success in legitimate ways?

The sure answer to that, dear reader, is the love of goodness for others and the sincere desire to positively influence their lives (the lives of many people).

That is, the person who would like to succeed in this way is certainly a great person in all the meaning of the word, and his heart is filled with many noble and moral values.

In order for you to understand my meaning well, dear reader, I will tell you the success story of Recep Tayyip Erdogan (the current President of Turkey), and this story is a good example of this kind of success.

This man (Recep Tayyip Erdogan) was born in 1956, in a poor neighbourhood in Istanbul.

After obtaining a doctorate degree (in economic sciences) from Marmara University in Turkey, he decided to engage in political work and joined a political party which was headed by Necmettin Erbakan.

After years of political work, Erdogan was able to rise further in that party, and in the political work in general (and becoming also Erbakan's best friend).

But this did not last long.

After a difference of opinion between Recep Erdogan and Necmettin Erbakan, Erdogan decided to withdraw from the Welfare Party (and from the Virtue Party, which was also headed by Necmettin Erbakan) and to establish his own party that reflects all his principles, ideas and perceptions that he had.

It is certainly the Justice and Development Party, the party that was destined to succeed in all the elections he faced (to this day) and which is currently ruling Turkey.

At first, Erdogan won in the Istanbul municipal elections (in 1994) and thus became mayor of the Turkish city, Istanbul.

Many of the residents of that city were not betting on him at the beginning, and they also doubted his ability (Erdogan) to fulfil the promises he made to them.

But contrary to all that, he made a great leap in that city.

In a short period of four years, he was able to pay off all the debts that had to be repaid, estimated at about $2 billion.

He even led it to become one of the most advanced cities in its region (and in the world as well).

Many facilities and infrastructure were built in it during that period (Erdogan's term) and also many world-class universities in addition to hospitals and sports spaces.

The Istanbul municipality has achieved incomes estimated at about four billion dollars during the term of Erdogan for that city.

All this happened in a short period of no more than four years. Recep Tayyip Erdogan has brought about great positive changes in that city, thanks to his rational policy and his good management of the resources it has (economic and human).

Thus, Istanbul became one of the cities that exemplify its great progress and prosperity, the thing that encouraged many to elect Erdogan as president of Turkey. This was actually achieved in the year 2003 when Recep Tayyip Erdogan was elected as the president of Turkey.

I think that everyone knows now the continuation of this story. Recep Tayyip Erdogan led Turkey towards economic growth and prosperity in all fields. Indeed, today it has become one of the most powerful countries in the world.

The per capita income has doubled during the Erdogan rule of 300%. The number of tourists visiting Turkey has also increased to about 40 million tourists annually, in addition to achieving a crude internal product estimated (annually) about 800 billion dollars and a financial reserve estimated at 114 billion dollars.

All these figures are the best evidence of Turkey's rise to the ranks of the world's major countries, unlike Escobar, who was motivated to succeed only by satisfying his pride and arrogance and extending his control and influence over others (dominating them).

Recep Erdogan would have liked to help his people and his countrymen and to lead Turkey on the path of success and prosperity in all its forms.

So, there is a big difference between Erdogan and Pablo Escobar. Erdogan is certainly one of the best presidents who passed all the history of Turkey, unlike Escobar, who can only be classified as a mere criminal who was behind the killing of many innocent people in Colombia and also smuggled tons of cocaine to various parts of the world.

So I hope, dear reader, that you do not try to succeed only in order to attract the attention (and admiration) of others to you and to satiate your pride, vanity and megalomania.

Because this will only lead you in the path of misery, and the end will be (definitely) catastrophic in every sense of the word.

If you want to be a successful person, try to be a great and positively influential person in your community and surroundings because that is what will enable you to get the precious thing called happiness.

So I invite you, dear reader, not to try to be successful and influential just to attract the attention and admiration of others (to you).

Wisdom
Part Three

Success which is intended only to arouse the attention and admiration of others, and to satisfy human pride and megalomaniac, is often acquired by illegal means. It also leads the person in the path to misery and unhappiness.

Positive and constructive success can only be achieved by a great person in all the meaning of the word, and the motivation behind this success is the moral and noble values that this person possesses in addition to his sincere desire to help others and influence them positively.

Chapter Four
You Are Already Rich

Perhaps the title of this paragraph seems a little bit provocative to you, dear reader. How can I know that you are rich or not? I don't know you personally and I don't even know your name, so how can I know that you are rich?

I know that you will wonder, dear reader, in this way (after reading the title of this part). This may seem strange to you, but it is not strange to me.

I will assure you once again that you are (really) rich.

I know that you live very richly, so I will explain it more clearly to you.

When I say that you are rich, I do not mean, dear reader, that you have more than a million dollars in your bank balance. After all, money is not the only criterion for wealth.

Wealth is something so much bigger than that, where money is only one of its aspects and only a small part of it.

Therefore, when a person does not have a large amount of money, this means that he is bankrupt and does not necessarily mean that he is poor. How can a person be described as poor when he has the blessings of hearing, sight, and speech (and walking and touching), and he lives on the surface of a planet that is considered one of the most beautiful planets in the universe, and the most capable to having the life of the human race, which is the Earth?

We are considered rich, whether we like it or not, because we have many blessings. Indeed, we cannot even count those blessings (from their abundance). We are really rich (and that's a fact).

Whatever your marital or financial situation, dear reader, it is advisable for you to not to ignore this fact.

I know that you would like to ask, dear reader, about the usefulness of this talk because having many blessings will not help you improve your financial situation, and it will not make any difference in your daily life. (I know that you will have this thinking while reading the previous lines). But I honestly not have the same opinion.

When a person pays attention to all the blessings that surround him, he will feel (certainly) gratitude and thanks, and he will also feel the great richness that he has in his life and in every moment of it, the thing that will bring him more blessings and will (also) generate more richness in his life.

Thanks and gratitude increase the blessings, and the person's sense of the great richness he has in his life also brings him more blessings.

Likewise, a person cannot live happily unless he feels that he is rich. Happiness is achieved only when a person feels rich in his life.

Also, when a person feels that he is happy, he attracts more happiness into his life.

Therefore, dear reader, you will not be happy in the future unless you live happily now; everything attracts its counterpart.

That mean, happiness attracts more happiness, and misery also attracts more misery.

So if you want to live happily in the future, you should be happy now. In order to be happy now, you must feel the many blessings that you receive and that life gives you, which you cannot even count them from their abundance.

Sensing these blessings is what makes you feel that you are rich, and your feeling that you are rich is what generates within you that true happiness and makes your heart spring with it.

If you feel that you are miserable, dear reader, it is likely that the source of that feeling is your focus only on the problems and difficulties that you suffer in your life and your disregard for all the blessings you enjoy.

In this context, I would also like to remind you, dear reader, that if you compare the blessings you have with the problems you suffer from, you will notice without any doubt that the problems do not even represent one of a 1000 when we compare them to the blessings that you have, and I am not exaggerating in my words.

In order to explain this to you further, I will insist you, dear reader, to imagine yourself living in a country other than your own and in circumstances that are completely different from yours.

Perhaps you expect me to talk to you about Somalia and the poverty in it, or about Ethiopia and the death of many citizens there due to starvation or malnutrition, or about the poor neighbourhoods of Mumbai and the degree of poverty and persecution experienced by the citizens there in addition to the large population that sometimes compels them to ride up trains and buses in order to move. Can you imagine that?

Or you expect me to tell you about the ghetto neighbourhoods in which many citizens live in the United States of America, where the trade of the cocaine and heroin is widespread and is the main source of income for the residents of those neighbourhoods in addition to the availability of weapons of all kinds and the constant fighting between them there. The thing that turned those neighbourhoods into hell for its residents.

No, I will not tell you about all this in order to prove the luxury that you enjoy, dear reader, in comparison with those places in this world of ours.

I will tell you about a much worse place. I will tell you about a country in which injustice and persecution are spreading to a degree that the world has never known before and has never been seen before. I will certainly talk to you, dear reader, about North Korea, the country of leader Kim Jong-un.

If I wanted to describe to you, dear reader, the leader of North Korea, Kim Jong-un, I would not find a more accurate description than his being a rare mixture of tyranny, arrogance and megalomania, a rare combination that can only be found in this person.

In order for you to understand my point well, dear reader, I will list some of the strangest and most repressive laws that do not exist in any other country but North Korea.

If, dear reader, you are in North Korea, and you want to watch an American movie or even just use the internet, (NB: there is no internet in North Korea because it is forbidden by the authorities) or just read a religious book (such as the Quran, the Bible or Tanakh), the penalty may be imposed on you. (There you get to the execution in the most brutal way).

It is done by a mortar (which is a cannon shell)!

That is, your corpse will be turned to pieces after the implementation of that unjust ruling against you.

Not only that but also that your parents and grandparents may also be executed because if someone breaks the law in North Korea, he and his entire family (that is, his parents and grandparents too) will be tried and punished. Can you imagine that!

You may find this strange and laughable as well, but there is something much stranger than that.

In 2015, Kim Jong-un executed the general engineer who oversaw the engineering and construction of Pyongyang International Airport because he did not like the airport design.

Kim and his wife had done a small tour on the international airport of Pyongyang. He did not like the design of the airport. So he executed the engineer of it.

This is not strange for a country like North Korea. Kim Jong-un had previously executed Former Defence Minister Hyun Yong Chol with an anti-aircraft gun because he slept during a military parade attended by North Korean leader (Kim Jong-un).

Thank God, dear reader, that you do not live in a country like North Korea, nor are you governed by a leader like Kim Jong-un! Otherwise, you would have also been executed with a mortar shell on charges of using the internet or watching an American movie.

We live in great blessings and in the most abundant of ages, so we should be grateful for all those blessings we have.

We are blessed with so many blessings that we cannot even count them (from their abundance).

So, dear reader, do not let the pressures and problems make you forget all that, and be thankful and grateful for all those blessings you enjoy because thanks and gratitude increase blessings.

But if you, dear reader, complain a lot, and are not satisfied with your life because you deserve better than what you get, then there are two possibilities.

The first possibility is to be honest about how you feel and that you really deserve a better life than the one you live.

In this case, complaining will not help you because what will really help you is that you seek to change yourself and your life for the better.

That is, to look for your mistakes and bad habits and then try to fix them while still striving for a real chance to save yourself from wasting your life.

Complaining will not help you in this case. What will really benefit you is to change yourself for the better by moving away from negative thoughts and bad habits and correcting the mistakes that you have previously committed in your life.

Complaining will not bring you the solution in this case, rather it will keep it away from you more.

Therefore, there is no benefit in complaining, dear reader, as it is one of the most destructive habits of human life. In other words, when you complain about your bad situation, you will make it worse.

Therefore, I invite you, dear reader, not to waste your time and energy with this destructive habit because it will definitely destroy your life if you take it as a habit (my passionate reader).

As for the second possibility, which is that you just have the illusion that you deserve a better life than the one you live, your situation is really difficult in this case. And I will not compliment you on this because doing so will push you into the abyss (and waste your life and your future as well).

And you should know in this case, dear reader that this illusion that you live in will give you a little comfort in the short term. But it will definitely destroy you in the long term.

Therefore, I hope from the bottom of my heart that you, dear reader, beware of being a prisoner of illusions and false beliefs that contradict the truth.

As for the habit of complaining that we are talking about, I sincerely hope that you will stay away from this destructive habit because it will only turn your difficult situation into a more difficult one.

As a summary of all of the above, I warn you, dear reader, that you shouldn't take complaint as a daily habit because it will certainly not help you change your life for the better.

What will benefit you is to live thankful for the blessings that you get every day and that life overflows you and also to strive changing yourself and your life in a positive way with your patience over the circumstances that you (may) be struggling now.

I know that you, dear reader, would like a realistic example that demonstrates the truthfulness of what I mentioned to you in the previous lines. Therefore, I will grant this request, and I will present to you the story of a poor Chinese young man who managed to escape from the difficult situation in which he was born and to become one of the richest people of his country and the world as well.

It is definitely the story of Jack Ma (founder of e-commerce website—Alibaba).

His story has turned him into an icon in the struggle and patience for failure until the time for success comes.

Jack Ma, who is ranked (currently) by Forbes magazine at number 34 in the list of the world's richest men, with an estimated fortune of about $22 billion, was not born with a silver spoon in his mouth.

On the contrary, it was a long journey of suffering and failure before he could finally achieve success.

He personally mentioned in one of the television interviews that he had failed three times in middle school in addition to his failure three other times to enter a university in China.

In fact, he had previously applied 30 times to work in small companies in China but was rejected in all of those jobs.

Do you know, dear reader, that Jack Ma, who is currently the richest man in China, once applied for work in KFC restaurant and 23 other people? He was the only one who was rejected (while all others persons have been accepted).

But this ambitious Chinese young man did not give up to despair, nor did he succumb under (the hard and the difficult) circumstances that he was constantly living in.

He was happy in spite of all what he had suffered in his life because he was certainly looking at the bright side of life, and he waited patiently for his opportunity, and he never wasted his energy complaining and indignant at his situation.

He was constantly striving to develop himself and take advantage of the previous mistakes he had made.

He repeatedly admitted that he was not good enough at this time, but he was also not resigned to his situation. Rather, he was constantly developing himself and benefitting from his previous mistakes.

Thus, after years of patience and not despair, the time for relief came for this Chinese man.

In 1999, Jack and his 18 friends launched the Alibaba website, which specialises in selling electronic products (in particular) via the internet (which is known as e-commerce).

Since then, Jack Ma's life has been flourishing to this day.

Alibaba has made big profits in the last ten years, which made Jack Ma rank today as the richest man in China.

This story is truly one of the most inspiring stories in the world, my dear reader, because if Jack Ma had not continued his constant patience over the many failures he faced in his life, he would not have been able to become today the richest man in China.

I would have found him to be a broken and unsuccessful person, mourning his misfortune and complaining about the difficulties and obstacles he faced in his life.

But Jack never did that.

After his long patience with the difficult circumstances he suffered in his life, he eventually discovered that he is one of the most fortunate people in this life.

He has managed to become the richest man in China and one of the richest men in the world as well.

His long patience and constant insight into the bright side of life are what made him transcend his difficult circumstances and become in the prestigious position he has now.

Jack always felt that he was rich even before he became a millionaire, as he was always looking at the blessings that surrounded him, the thing that made him a happy person (even before he became financially rich).

If Jack had been so focused on his constant and permanent failure that he had previously suffered, he would become a failure, unable to help even himself. He would have been crazy or had committed suicide if he had done so.

But he never did that. He kept rejoicing in life and looking at its bright side. This enabled him to overcome the difficult circumstance that he was suffering from and also made him the richest man in China after that.

Focusing on the bright side of life generates in the person a sense of gratitude. And gratitude increases blessings and brings wealth in all its forms.

Therefore, I wish you, dear reader, to not see the problems and difficulties that you suffer from in your life and to live gratefully and thankfully for all the blessings that life overflows to you and which you cannot even count from their abundance (such as health, food and drinks, etc.).

You are already rich, dear reader.

Wisdom
Part Four

Your focus on the many blessings you enjoy (which you cannot even count) generates in you, dear reader, feelings of gratitude and thanks. And thanks with the gratitude increases the blessings (which the person has).

Every human being on the Earth is considered rich because he has many and many blessings. Richness can never be reduced into just the material dimension.

Chapter Five
Don't Resist Life Changes if You Want to Be Happy

Yes, dear reader, do not resist the changes and vicissitudes of life to not be in misery.

Change is one of the ways of life (and the universe as well), so everything changes in this life, especially in our time (where everything is changing quickly).

Therefore, there is no reason to resist life changes or try to escape from them because life is changing in all times.

Everything changes in this life, and even our external appearance also changes (our shape, weight, height…).

Change is one of the ways of life and one of its (permanent) characteristics.

Everything, dear reader, in this life is constantly changing.

Thus, the person who is considered intelligent is certainly the person who adapts to the changes and vicissitudes of life. He does not try to collide with it or resist it (and not keep going with it). This person is well aware that change is one of the eternal laws of this life—and one of its permanent characteristics.

Therefore, I wish you, dear reader, to be clever in dealing with life's changes and constant fluctuations and not to try to clash or conflict with it because doing so will make you the loser in the end.

A person who is considered intelligent is certainly a person who has flexibility and good adaptability to change because if every person does not do this, he will lead his life to destruction and loss in the end.

I know that you would like to ask now, dear reader, why so many people resist change in all its forms. What are the hidden reasons? Why so many people resist the changes and vicissitudes of life?

The sure reason for this, dear reader, is fear (in all its forms). Many people resist change because they think it will cause them failure, loneliness or even financial problems. They are afraid that change will cause them suffering and pain in all its forms.

So, the question we must ask is: Does change really cause us suffering and pain?

To answer this question, I will present to you, dear reader, my personal view of the change and the impact it can make in the person's life.

From my humble opinion, dear reader, change may cause you some suffering and problems at first.

But it will lead you in the end towards a better life than you were living (before it happened).

That is, all these problems and difficulties are only a test and scrutiny for you. Change is what reveals to us the nature of each person and shows us his truth.

When the conditions of a particular person change for the worse, we can know what is his reality and his inner strength as well. The strongest people are also the most afflicted.

That's mean. A strong person is the one who is patient with the bad changes that may occur to him in his life, and at the same time, he also struggles to overcome those difficulties (which he may be exposed to in his life).

I know that these previous lines may be somewhat difficult for you to understand, dear reader. So I will tell you the success story of Wallace Johnson (founder of the Holiday Inn chain).

This story is considered one of the most inspiring stories in the world about the impact of man's adaptation to the negative changes that may occur to him in his life in determining his fate and future as well.

In 1942, Wallace Johnson was working as a carpenter in an American company specialising in building homes where Wallace Johnson was a skilled craftsman in making wooden floors for homes (NB: In America, the floors of homes are made of wood, and Wallace Johnson's role in that company was to build that floor).

Johnson was an ordinary man like everyone else, working for a monthly salary of a few dollars, and he was from the middle class in America (at that time).

He lived a normal life, and he also owned a house and supported his small family consisting of his wife and his children.

But in that fateful year (in the year 1942), a major and stifling financial crisis occurred for the company in which he was working, forcing them to lay off some employees in order to reduce expenses.

Hence, the choice fell on Wallace Johnson (also), and they decided to dispense with him, even though he had worked with them for nearly 20 years.

This decision was a real shock to Wallace Johnson. After all the work he made in that company and sacrificing his effort and time for 20 years, his reward in the end was his dismissal and dispensation from working in it.

This was very cruel to this American man.

So imagine, dear reader, that you will be dismissed from a company you worked for all that time. It is a cruel and bitter thing in every sense of the word.

Any person this will happen to him expected that he will suffer a great depression, and after that, he will live his life in a great sadness and unhappiness and he may even turn into a negative person who is constantly complaining and destructive, and he is completely losing the hope in this life.

But Wallace Johnson was not. He decided to face this harsh event with great strength and steadfastness.

After suffering from unemployment (for a short period), he decided to mortgage his (only) house that he owned, and with the money he would get from that mortgage, he decided to establish a small company to build houses.

This was shocking (really) to both his wife and his children's because if Wallace Johnson failed to run the small company he founded, they would suffer homelessness.

But his wife encouraged him in the end to do so—because she believed in him—and was fully aware of the great experience that her husband had accumulated in the field of building houses, which he gained through his work in that company for 20 years.

Indeed, Wallace Johnson began working in the field of building small and medium-sized houses in Memphis (southern USA) in 1942.

After Wallace Johnson built two small houses (after setting up his own small business), he was able to get his mortgage back (with which he had mortgaged his house), which encouraged him to continue with that business.

Indeed, Wallace Johnson continued to work in this field for nearly 10 years. He earned a huge fortune that enabled him to invest in the hotel business.

After building several hotels in the United States of America, Wallace Johnson was able to establish his own brand, which is called today the Holiday Inn, which is a chain of high-quality hotels (which are now present in various parts of the world).

Thus, Wallace Johnson became one of the richest people in the world, as the Holiday Inn chain of hotels is considered one of the biggest hotel chains in our world today.

Wallace Johnson has a famous phrase he always says: "I would like to thank the director of the company who fired me from the work in his company."

If the economic conditions of that company had not changed (to the worse), Wallace Johnson would not have been fired from working for it, and he would not have been able to become one of the richest people in America and the world as well.

Change, dear reader, is one of the laws of life and one of its important laws.

But the important thing that makes a difference in a person's life is not the change itself. Rather, it is the extent to which a person adapts and accepts change (that is, the extent to which he accepts the changes and fluctuations of life that occur constantly). Everything is in constant change in this life (which we live).

Therefore, a person who does not want any change in his life, and wants to live in permanent stability throughout his life, is definitely a person ignorant of the laws and rules of life, which will make him automatically lead his life towards destruction and loss.

Change is one of the laws of life and one of the laws of the universe.

Therefore, the person who does not adapt to change will lead himself towards loss as well as destruction.

If Wallace Johnson had not adapted to the tragic accident that he suffered, which is his dismissal from work (at the age of 40), he would not have become one of the richest men in the world, and he would not have established the Holiday Inn chain of hotels, which is currently considered one of the biggest hotel chains in the world (and one of the best).

If Wallace Johnson chose not to adapt to change and to become a person resentful of himself and his society and constantly complained about the injustice he had been subjected to (which is represented in his expulsion from that company after working for it nearly 20 years ago), you would have found him after that as a failed and destructive human being who could not benefit even himself (and may also become a burden on himself and on his society).

But Wallace Johnson adapted to the injustice he was subjected to and decided to face life and did not try to hide from it.

So he didn't blame himself, his family (and his society) or the US government for not helping him in his difficult situation (which he was living in at that time).

Wallace Johnson decided to take that injustice that he was subjected to as something that strengthened him and gave him a great incentive to work and proved himself and his presence in this life (and also benefit from the experiences he had accumulated in the field of building houses, in which he had worked for nearly 20 years).

Thus, Wallace Johnson transformed the painful event of his dismissal into a big positive energy that drove him to work with greater diligence and dedication, which made him one of the richest men in USA.

So he doesn't blame the American government and demand that it compensated him and gave him a sum of money (on a monthly basis) so that he could live with it.

He became the one who gave the US government money by paying taxes estimated annually in the millions of dollars.

After that, Wallace Johnson lived his life in luxury, enjoying whatever he wanted in the life. (It is truly one of the most inspiring stories in the world, dear reader).

After that, Wallace Johnson died in 1988. He died and he is considered one of the richest people in the world, and he was the owner of the Holiday Inn chain of hotels (famous in the whole world) which owned more than half of its market value, which is estimated today in billions of dollars.

I think that this beautiful and realistic story that I told you, dear reader, is the best evidence that when a person does not lose hope in life and maintains his positivity, optimism and good faith in God Almighty, he will eventually be able to overcome all his failures and bad stations. (And he will also overcome all the negative changes that may occur to him in his life).

Wallace Johnson maintained his positivity, his good faith and his optimism for life despite the harshness of what he was exposed to. Thus, in the end, he managed to succeed and get everything he dreamt about in this life.

Many people may think that success is nothing more than luck.

That is, all successful people in this world are only lucky, unlike people who suffer in this life, because their suffering is due to their luck and misfortune.

But all this is nothing more than nonsense. This saying has a great detraction from the value of successful people. There is no such thing in this life as what we called luck.

But there is the god-giving.

A positive and good-natured person who wishes to positively influence his society cannot, of course, be lost by God's mercy.

Luck is not believed by successful people in this life but only by broken and unsuccessful people (in order to justify their hatred and envy against successful people).

There is no such thing as luck. Rather, there is a giving from God.

Wallace Johnson, despite the cruelty of what happened to him in his life, has maintained his positivity, optimism and good faith in this life, and he did not become (also) a resentful and envious person, as he did not hate those who expelled him.

Rather, he made that painful event that he was exposed to a source of his strength (and great energy) which he used to unload in his work.

So he tried to not be resentful, envious and hateful of his society, and he chose not to go that way at all.

Rather, he chose to transform himself into a constructive (and productive) energy to his society.

Thus, through his hard work (and sincerity in his work), he was able to become one of the richest people in the world (and one of the top businessmen as well).

So we can derive one meaning from this story, which is that when a person adapts to the changes that occur in his life (even if they are very terrible and bad), he will eventually reach a much better life (than the one he was living before the events occurred).

Change is one of the ways of life, and one of the laws of the universe, so there is no way to escape from it. There is only one solution, which is to adapt to it and keep pace with it and to maintain positivity, optimism and good faith in life.

The thing that will make us discover in the end is that this change was in our favour, as it has led us to a life much better than the one we lived before it occurred, or the one we would have lived without it happening.

So, adapting to change is the only option available to us in this life because we are simply the ones who generate those changes in it.

If you want to become a millionaire, they will certainly fire you from your job (as happened with Wallace Johnson), and you will suffer two things in the beginning (problems and obstacles that you did not consider) which are preparing you for the life you want to live.

In the end, if you adapt to that change (which you attracted to your life through your thoughts) and also believe in yourself, then you will be able to live that life that you dream about.

We, dear reader, attract change into our lives through our thoughts.

God wants us to live that life that we want and dream about, so changes happen every day (and in every hour too) in this life.

Because it is simply a compass that leads us towards that life that we want to live.

So there is no way to object to it (or try to resist life changes). Because who does that will end up losing and destroying himself.

Perhaps, dear reader, you would like a good example (which explains this further).

So I will tell you (also) the most prominent story of not keeping pace with change in our current time (since the beginning of the new millennium). It is certainly the story of Nokia.

This giant company, which was considered only in the year 2006 as one of the most prominent multinational companies in the field of manufacturing and selling high-quality mobile phones.

Nokia… if there is a description by which we can describe its products (and mobile phones), it is certainly the high quality (in the manufacturing process).

So what happened to Nokia? And why did it completely disappear from the mobile phone market in 2014?

And why it declared bankruptcy and was unable to compete the mobile phone companies presenting in the market now? (Despite being classified only in 2006 as a giant company in the world of manufacturing of mobile phones, and it was far superior to all other companies that are still present).

So why did Nokia collapse so quickly despite having achieved only in the year 2007 transactions of more than 50 billion dollars (and a net profit estimated at 13 billion dollars)?

So what happened to Nokia? Why did it lose its market value so quickly?

Only in 2006, Nokia sold more than a quarter of a billion phones of its high-quality mobile phones. (Nb: Nokia phone is impossible to break; it is designed to be so strong to shocks).

So what's happened to that giant company (Nokia)?

What led to the decline in its market value and its disappearance in the beginning of 2014?

The story, dear reader, can be summed up in one phrase, which is: Change is one of life's rules, and one of its laws, and every person who does not adapt to change will be fade at the end (even if it is gradually).

So the story, dear reader, is that in the year 2007, a major change occurred in the world of mobile phones, which is that Apple manufactured a phone that can be also connected with the internet service (iPhone).

That is, Apple's phones also provide a service for browsing the internet websites in addition to the ability of its users to access the most popular and widespread applications in the world at that time (and in these days also), like YouTube, Facebook, Messenger and other applications that were popular and widely spread in that time.

Consequently, there were aspects of a major change that would be occurring in the world of mobile phones, as its function would no longer be limited to just enabling the user to communicate with others (for example: one's family and friends).

No, mobile phones will become like small computers. Its users can browse (through it) all websites and webpages in addition to enabling them to access all social networking sites through the android system on which these mobile phones are available (or iOS the system of the iPhones) which enables users of these mobile phones to access the internet service.

All those working in the field of communication were confirming the use of the android system (which is free and available for all companies).

However, Nokia didn't want to include this technology in its mobile phones, as it did not want to keep pace with these new techniques that appeared in the world of communication.

And it was betting on Symbian, through which it was able to sell billions of its products around the world (which enabled it to become one of the largest companies in the field of mobile phones' manufacturing).

Therefore, Nokia, unlike all other companies that work in the field of communication (which all chose the android system), it preferred to bet on the Symbian operating system through which it was able to achieve its previous successes.

In other words, Nokia was betting on its previous successes (and on its long history in the field of manufacturing mobile phones) and also on the great market value that it had at that time.

However, that never worked for this company. Rather, it was what led this company towards destruction and eventual loss (and the total disappearance from the mobile phone market by 2014).

Nokia was sold to Microsoft for an estimated $7.2 billion dollars.

This was the end of Nokia. This company whose products benefitted millions of people on the surface of this Earth and to which everyone attests to the quality of its products and the length of their validity (time of use). It was known that the Nokia mobile phone was the phone that did not crash.

But it is unfortunate, dear reader, that Nokia is the one that crashed in 2014.

And the reason, of course, is that it did not adapt with the change that took place in the world of mobile phones in the year 2007.

Each writer has his own point of view and his unique angle from which he looks at the events, alterations and changes that occur in life.

As for me, I firmly believe that if a person does not keep pace with the changes that occur in the world and keep pace with them, then he will disappear, fade and eventually get loss.

Thus, the mistake that killed Nokia, from my personal (and humble) point of view, is certainly its failure to keep pace with the change that occurred in the world of mobile phones, represented by the emergence of the android system (which enables mobile phones to access the internet service and also browse pages, applications and social media sites) where mobile phones have become small computers.

All customers and users of Nokia phones were expecting this company to provide them with this system (android operating system).

However, Nokia disappointed the expectations of all its users and decided to keep the Symbian system (which is very weak when we compare it to the android system).

That was the reason for the destruction of Nokia and its disappearance from the world of mobile phones.

Since the advent of that service (the android operating system), Nokia has incurred daily losses estimated at about $23 million.

As everyone stood in a state of astonishment and wonder why Nokia did not use the android system (although it is free and available to all companies).

The reason is quite simple, dear reader. It is the attachment of Nokia to its golden era (the eighties and nineties of the last century) which were like the honeymoon for this company, as it was able through its use of the Symbian (system) to achieve annual revenues estimated at billions of dollars.

It was those years that made Nokia's strength, which also contributed to its market value reaching $90 billion in 2007.

But life is not in stability and constancy, but in continuous and permanent change, and everyone who does not keep pace with that development and change disappears with time.

Perhaps the story of Nokia is the best proof of that.

The company that was considered dominant in the mobile phones' market (just at the beginning of the new millennium) has disappeared today.

Only because it did not keep pace with the change that took place in 2007 and did not use the new technology that appeared (which is the system android).

So, the summary of this part, dear reader (and the lesson learnt from it) is that change is one of the laws of life and one of its (immutable) laws.

There is no way for resisting change or trying to escape from it because that will only lead the person in the path of misery, material and moral loss also.

Change is the only thing that remains constant in this life, and that does not change with the passage of time.

Life is ever-changing since its beginning. All previous populations believed in change, and that it is one of the constants and norms of life that do not change (over time).

Therefore, the main lesson that I would like to give you in this part is that when a person adapts and accepts the changes that are constantly occurring in his life, he leads himself towards a better life than the one he was living before the occurrence of these changes.

That is, he leads himself on the path of happiness and success in all its forms (as happened in the story of the American businessman—Wallace Johnson—and his impressive success in the hotel field after accepting that he was fired from the company that he worked for (nearly a 20 years).

And in the case that a person wants to resist the changes of the life and do not adapt to them, he will lead himself in the path of misery. He will only destroy himself in the end.

You will disappear with time (as happened with Nokia when it decided not to use the android system, it completely disappeared a few years after the appearance of that application, despite it being a company that everyone witnessed for its high quality in manufacturing its products, durability and long life. Who have these products, despite all the advantages that this company possess, it has completely disappeared from the mobile phone market since the year 2014).

So it is better for you, dear reader, to adapt to all the changes that occur in your life.

Even if these changes seem to you negative and very terrible, they will eventually lead you toward a better life than the one you were living before the occurrence of these events and changes.

Do not forget, dear reader, that every great human he has been exposed to many negative situations and changes in his life, and he was able, after adapting to them and accepting them, to live at the end a better life than the one he had before the occurrence of these changes.

Adapting to the negative changes that may occur in a man's life, and also being patient with the difficult circumstances that may result from them, always leads a person to a better life than the one he was living (before the occurrence of these negative bad changes).

So I hope that you, dear reader, will not forget that, and that you will always adapt to the changes and fluctuations that may occur in your life because change is one of the laws of life and one of its constant laws. So I hope that you will not forget that.

Wisdom
Part Five

Adapting to change leads a person to live a better life than the one he was living before it occurred. A person's failure to adapt to change leads him to gradual decline and loss.

Change is one of the laws of life, and one of its constants facts, so everything changes in this life (from economic conditions to living conditions...). Everything is in continuous change in this life, the thing that makes adapting to change and keeping pace with it a necessity, and not only an available option for the person (everyone must adapt to the changes and fluctuations of life, and he has no other choice; if he does not, doing so will cause him to disappear and lose his path.

A person is the one who attracts change to himself because when the person wants to rise more his standard of living or in his financial situation, it is certain that many changes will happen to him, which can be seen as a negative thing in the short term. But it is considered as a preparation for him so that he can live after that (in the long term) the life that he dreams about.

Chapter Six
You Are Not Your Mind

Yes (my dear reader), you are not your mind, and you can never reduce your being in just your mind. The mind is nothing but a biological organ, so how could you be your mind?

You are an entity and a soul that God provided with a heart and a body.

This body contains the mind, whose role is limited to being a storehouse of ideas, events and situations that a person has previously experienced or seen in his life, something that helps him during the thinking process.

That is, the role of the mind is represented in being an assistant in the thinking process.

That is, it is not he who thinks but you who think with his help.

Thus, the body is nothing but a vessel for the soul, spirit and heart, a vessel that helps you to live on this Earth and to satisfy all your needs that require your physical presence (such as work, eating, sleeping and procreation).

So you are a soul equipped with a heart and a body.

The function of this last trio (comprised of the spirit, heart and body) is helping you live properly and to remain in constant contact with the society in which you live and with the spirit of the world as well.

Therefore, when you think that you are your mind, you are not only committing spiritual suicide, but in many cases, this may lead to absolute madness. It could also be the cause of your unhappiness.

Do not, then, dear reader, attach yourself to your mind because you will make yourself a prisoner to your mind.

The mind is nothing but a tool that helps you to think properly and to benefit (also) from the experiences and situations that you have gone through before.

But the tragedy that many people suffer from today is represented in making the mind a prison for themselves.

Consequently, as a result of that, you find many people doing many negative and immoral behaviours and actions which do not represent them and do not embody their truth or character but only represent what they have previously witnessed in their lives.

You will find (for example) that the husband beats his wife only because he had previously witnessed his father beating his mother. Therefore, he involuntarily imitates that despite the fact that he is not convinced by that.

And herein comes the danger. When a man becomes a slave to his mind, he will find himself doing many actions and behaviours that he does not want to do.

You will find, for example, that many young men have become drug addicts only because they have previously seen their friends do so, or that many girls have become involved in prostitution only because they have seen their best friends do that.

And all of this has one (and only) source, which is the connection of the soul with the mind, or in a more accurate sense, the slavery of man to his mind.

When a person is connected to his mind, he subconsciously imitates everything he sees in his surroundings, which leads him (in many cases) to do many deviant and heinous acts, which not reflect him (or his morals).

In order to summarise all of the above, I find no good in the statement that the mind is a good tool, but it is a corrupt master.

Beware, dear reader, of making him a master of you because he will lead you into his dark prison.

And if this happens and you are afflicted with this, then all you have to do to escape from that prison is to search for your truth and your essence, as disengaging from your mind is only through knowing yourself well. (It can benefit in this case of practicing some spiritual activities such as meditation, for example).

So I invite you, dear reader, to not fall into that dark trap because it will only lead you in the path of misery and sadness.

Your association with your mind may be, dear reader, the cause of your misery and difficult living conditions.

Rather, this can also expose you to many serious mental illnesses or even suicide and sheer madness.

In order for you to understand this well, I will tell you, dear reader, the story of a famous German philosopher in the late 19th century, but he lived a gloomy and miserable life, and he also suffered a nervous breakdown (in the last years of his life). He is certainly the famous German philosopher Friedrich Nietzsche.

Friedrich Nietzsche, who is considered one of the most prominent philosophers, was known for his great intelligence and his ability to analyse and see behind the lines.

He was able, with his fervent thought and great enthusiasm, to dive deeply and with great thought into the deep dimensions that human behaviour means.

No one can deny that Nietzsche was one of the most prominent philosophers of his prime. His principles and ideas had a great impact on major world leaders in the middle of the last century, such as Hitler and Mussolini.

Hitler once gifted Mussolini one of Friedrich Nietzsche's books in a clear and explicit reference to the great position that German philosopher had.

But if you decide one day (dear reader) to read one of Friedrich Nietzsche's writings or books, or even to read, for example, his most famous book—*Thus Spoke Zarathustra*, without a doubt, you will stand amazed and shocked at the difficulties of understand its meanings.

If this book indicates something, it indicates that it came out of the mind of a sick and arrogant person who contradicts himself so much.

Rather, he is about to go mad from the intensity of his contradictions.

Friedrich Nietzsche was one of the fiercest opponents of noble principles and morals.

As this deranged philosopher supported the execution of the weak, the poor and those with congenital defects (who suffer from deformities and physical diseases).

He also hated the poor so much and despised them.

And he was expressing his dissatisfaction with the forms of injustice and suffering that prevailed among people.

And another time completely contradicts himself and says that the law of power must prevail. That is, it is the predominance of the strongest, and the strong man should be ruling the weak as he wants and even to kill them as well (kill or rape their women).

If I am stronger than you financially, physically or intellectually, for example, then I have the right to apply all forms of oppression on you and to humiliate you as well.

But the strange thing about all of this is that Nietzsche himself was not physically fine. He suffered throughout his life from syphilis, which worsened to make him a (semi-permanent-feeling) headache. Hence, he was also weak physically.

Nietzsche's disadvantages did not end. He also hated all the religions in addition to his intense hatred of religious people in all their forms.

Therefore, Nietzsche was following whatever he liked and he believed in any foolishness that crossed his mind. He was following whatever his mind dictated to him without the slightest distinction of what is right and what is not right.

He utters any foolishness that his mind dictated to him. Rather, he believed in it as well, and was hostile to everyone who disagreed with him in opinion or intellectual orientation without the slightest doubt in his opinion which he was convinced of.

Every word he uttered, he considered correct no matter how true and credible it was.

Thus, after years of that deviant lifestyle that Nietzsche lived, which was full of arrogance, and utter paranoia,

Nietzsche suffered a nervous breakdown in the year 1889, and he entered, at the age of 44, a mental hospital after he was completely insane and he became a psychopath (officially).

This happened after he was seen dancing naked in a street in the Italian city of Turin, in addition to causing chaos in a school and thinking of killing the governor as well.

So, this sad story that Friedrich Nietzsche lived clearly embodies, dear reader, an important truth, which is: The mind is a good tool but is a corrupt master.

When a person makes his mind a master over him (as the German philosopher Friedrich Nietzsche did), he will certainly do many acts and behaviours, which in many cases are disgraceful, immoral and illegal also.

Rather, it is contrary to the truth and essence of man.

Therefore, I invite you, dear reader, to discover yourself well and not to make your mind as your master, as it will lure you little by little to fall into the depression and stress by motivating you to constantly think about the problems and difficulties that you suffer from at your life, which will make it worse. Your constant thinking about problems will make you a complainant, which will lead you committing many mistakes and foolishness and thus will multiply your problems.

Therefore, I repeat my warning to you, dear reader, against swimming in that dirty swamp because overthinking in problems will only lead to their exacerbation.

Your constant thinking will not help you in obtaining a solution to the problems that you suffer from.

What will help you in this is to search for a realistic and right solution to it and making the right decisions.

As for the thing that can help you in that, it is certainly your intuition and your inner feeling that comes to you from your heart.

So, if you, dear reader, are suffering from a problem, then I hope that you will maintain your positive attitudes and your good faith in God.

Because that is what will stimulate your intuition, and it will also help you reach the solution quickly.

But that will not come to you unless your heart is full of principles, morals and positive constructive values.

So, the main thing that a person should pay attention to and be cautious to fill it with positive values is certainly his heart.

It is the spiritual heart of a person that inspires him to the correct and right path that he should follow.

Because it is the spiritual heart of a person that is considered the link between him and his Creator.

In order for you to understand this well, dear reader, I will tell you a story that took place in Nepal (which is a neighbouring region of India) and is also famous for being the birthplace of the great philosopher who is considered one of the greatest philosophers throughout history. He is certainly Siddhartha Gautama—nicknamed Buddha.

In the year 560 BCE, the world was on a date with the birth of one of the greatest philosophers of all time.

In the Himalayas, specifically in the Nepal region, the ruler of Shakya was waiting for the birth of his son, Siddhartha Gautama.

It was an absolutely extraordinary event. In addition to embodying the date of birth of the son of the king of the

Shakya region of Nepal, the child Siddhartha himself was not an ordinary child.

When his father used the priests of the palace to predict the future of the little prince, the priests were amazed when they noticed 32 signs on the body of the child, Siddhartha, which indicated that he would either become a great military emperor or he would become one of the great sages of his time.

His father rejoiced with great joy, as he wished himself that his son would become a great military emperor and rule all the regions of the country that he was unable to rule.

But on the other hand, he was most afraid that his son, Siddhartha Gautama, would become wise.

In order to keep him away from thinking about the wisdom and the deep meanings of life, he provided all material pleasures to his son, Siddhartha, so that he could not think about anything.

Child Siddhartha grew up surrounded by all the pleasures and entertainments.

His father had ordered his every whim to be fulfilled, and thus this prince had everything he wanted in his life, starting with the best types of food to the most beautiful clothes and jewels in addition to gold and money and ending with wine and the most beautiful women of his country.

But the strangest thing in this story, dear reader, is that the Prince Siddhartha Gautama, despite enjoying everything he liked, remained a miserable young man with gloomy features, and he did not live a happy day in his father's palace despite all that he had.

And the days passed, until that day came when Prince Siddhartha decided to abandon his father's palace, leaving behind all that great bliss.

This seemed insane to everyone in the palace.

So why did Prince Siddhartha Gautama decide to leave all that great bliss in which he was living and embarked on a journey into the unknown?

So, everyone who was in that palace wondered with astonishment about him.

However, the reason is simple—the prince's unwillingness to be a military emperor because that did not like what he loved and aspired to do.

Siddhartha Gautama was always contemplating and thinking about wisdom and the deep meanings of life and about sublime principles and values (too).

So he never loved the palace life despite all the luxury and bliss he enjoyed.

Therefore, he set out with some of his faithful servants on a journey of self-discovering (which was undertaken by that prince).

During that trip, Siddhartha was perpetuating meditation and ancient Indian rituals that help a person to know himself more.

And he was also, at the beginning, living with (extreme) austerity, not eating much food and avoiding all material pleasures (and all forms of luxury as well) until this prince became a lean body and weak. Rather, he was about to perish from the excessive malnutrition he was suffering from.

Here, the prince discovered that like a person suffers from life that revolves only around luxury and momentary pleasures, he also suffers when he avoids all material and luxury means.

Thus, the wise prince concluded that a person should be balanced in his dealings with material things and that it is good to possess them but it is bad to attach himself to them.

And so the days passed, and Prince Siddhartha continued to meditate moderately every day in addition to learning all the ancient wisdoms that help a person to live a positive and healthy (and constructive) life.

A few years later, Prince Siddhartha Gautama became very wise and became dubbed as Buddha (the enlightened), as he became one of the great philosophers and sages of his time.

He was very famous in many Asian countries such as India, Nepal and China.

Since people, out of their great respect and love for him, considered him as a god, despite his denunciation of that. (NB: I am not promoting the Buddhist religion through this book, but rather I am telling you the true story of Buddha, who is considered as one of the most prominent philosophers and wise men of all time).

So this, dear reader, was the story of the famous philosopher Siddhartha Gautama (Buddha).

And this inspiring story is the best proof that when a person follows his intuition and his inner feeling (which God gives him), he would be able to live in true happiness that it comes from the depth of his heart.

Buddha (for example) followed his heart, his intuition and his inner sense, so he fled from his father's palace which provided him with all material pleasures, and the reason is certainly that he did not find himself.

He did not even live a happy day in his father's palace.

He did not want to become an emperor or a military commander, but rather he liked to practice meditation and wanted to search for wisdom and the deep meanings of life.

Thus, after years of suffering and problems that the young prince was exposed to (after leaving his father's palace), he was finally able to win and overcome them.

Prince Siddhartha has come to be considered as one of the great sages of his time (if he was not actually the greatest sage of his time) and after that, he became of high importance and of value and an important influencer (in his time).

He even managed to become rich—and richer than his father (who became proud of him).

And he lived after that in happiness and bliss until his death.

So (dear reader), when a person follows his heart, he can live in true happiness. The spiritual heart is the true source of happiness.

That is, a person cannot be happy while he is in conflict with his heart.

But the problem that many people face and that hinders them from following their heart is that the heart may lead a person to many problems and difficulties.

But I will assure you, dear reader, that all these problems are only at the beginning, and they can be considered as an exam and a test of human toughness.

So the person who truly follows his heart will eventually be able to overcome those problems and (also) reach the life he dreams of.

Buddha (for example) was able after following his heart, and after facing the problems and difficulties that befell him at the beginning, to reach the life he dreamt of (that he wanted to live).

And not only Buddha but also all people who are happy and successful in their lives have followed their heart and their inner sense.

Many people may think that it is madness for a person to follow his heart.

But this is nothing more than nonsense; most of the people who are successful and happy and who positively influence their society have followed their heart.

And if a person does not do this, he will become a negative thinker, and he will gradually lead his life to the path of destruction.

Rather, he may go crazy in the end, as happened with the famous German philosopher Friedrich Nietzsche, and as it also happens with many people who suffer from mental or chronic mental illnesses.

All of this has one source, which is the abundance of negative thinking, and the person's following of everything that crosses his mind (or in a more accurate sense, the slavery of a person to his mind).

Beware, dear reader, of following everything that comes to your mind because the mind is a good tool, but it is a corrupt master.

So following a person to his heart is the source of all positive and constructive actions and a source of happiness and success as well.

As for following the person, his mind (and neglecting his inner intuition), is the factor that generates all the misery that people suffer in our world today.

I wish you, dear reader, that you follow your heart.

This (also) does not mean that you neglect your mind; the mind is a good tool. Beware, dear reader, of making him your master because it will only lead you to the misery.

As conclusion, dear reader, you are not your mind.

Wisdom
Part Six

A person's following of his mind leads him towards negative thinking in all its forms. And the abundance of negative thinking is considered the main source of depression, unhappiness and misery—and even psychological and neurological diseases. A person's slavery to his mind is one of the most destructive things to him because the mind is a good tool but is a corrupt master.

A person's attainment of happiness and the life he dreams of is related to the extent to which he follows his inner feeling and his heart. The path of the heart is the path of happiness.

Chapter Seven
At the End, You Will Die and (Me Too) ...

In the year 1985, on the slopes of the Andes Mountains, Mountain Climber Joe Simpson and his friend Simon Yates were preparing to climb Mount Siula Grande (which reaches a height of about 6500 metres) to become the first climbers to climb that huge mountain (which is located in Peru).

The young English climber Joe Simpson (Joe and his friend Simon are actually considered the first to climb that mountain) was surprised during his descent (from the top of that mountain) that he suffered a serious fracture in his right ankle.

This was very dangerous because when a mountain climber breaks one of his ankles, it simply means certain death.

His friend (Simon) really wanted to help him get off the top of that mountain.

But without success, after that Joe Simpson had another accident. (He fell into a snow crack from a height of 50 meters). It was a fatal accident in every sense of the word.

But there was a bigger problem, which was that Simon had lost the rope that connected him to Joe Simpson, so he could no longer help his friend (Simpson).

So he came down from that mountain alone (without Joe Simpson) because he thought he had died after falling from that high altitude (which was estimated at 50 metres).

Then Joe Simpson woke up from his coma and found himself alone in that snowy crack.

But after a long search, he found a way out of that rift and was able to go out to the surface of that mountain.

Then he continued his crawl in order to reach the bottom (the bottom of the mountain).

After a few days had passed, Joe was actually able to come down from that mountain.

Fortunately, he found his friend (Simon) still in the camp they had set up at the bottom of the mountain (because he was thinking that his friend Joe had died, so he could not leave the camp).

Simon then transferred his friend (Joe Simpson) into hospital for healing.

And all hope was that Joe Simpson would survive.

He was subjected to a fatal accident, and therefore, his survival (even if he was permanently disabled) was a real miracle.

But the strange thing about this English climber's story is that he was able to recover fully after only two years of that accident.

It was really unbelievable. After 24 months, Simpson was able to live like any normal person, as if nothing had happened.

He began to walk on his feet naturally, as if his fall was just an imagination.

And today, he is still alive and in full physical and mental strength (thanks to God).

There is no logical or scientific explanation why the English climber did not die, except that the power of God made him continue to live. (Any person would fall from a height of 50 meters, from the top of one of the largest mountains in the world, he will certainly die, but Joe Simpson survived that however).

He has the chance to live after that accident, and today he is still in full mental and physical strength.

I think you have understood, dear reader, the significance of this story that I have just told you.

Your age, dear reader, is written, and it will not decrease or increase even by one second. When the time comes for your departure from this world, you will leave, dear reader.

So it is important for you, dear reader, to prepare yourself well for this day because sooner or later, you will die and leave this world.

I know that you, dear reader, would like to wonder about the nature of that world to which we will all leave after our death.

Is there really another life after death?

Or in other words, could not all those hadiths that are narrated about the transition to the other world (after death) be mere myths? Can we become nothing after our death?

The answer to all these questions is simple, dear reader. A person is a soul (or an entity), meaning that each of the soul, heart and body are nothing but tools that God has provided us to the reason that we can live normally and so that we can also perform our tasks.

That means that the body is nothing but a tool that helps us live on the surface of this planet and also enables us to practice our natural activities, such as work, eating, drinking or procreation (and the body also represents our physical dimension).

Thus, the body with all its organs is nothing but a tool that God has given to us in order to serve us to live well.

Thus, death is nothing but a separation from the body. That is, when a person dies, he is separated from his body, and he also moves from the physical dimension to the spiritual dimension.

That is, death is nothing but the annihilation of the body and the transition of man to the world of spirits.

I know that you would like to ask, dear reader, about the nature of this other world (the world of spirits) to which we will all move after our death.

In order to answer, dear reader, this important question will come to your mind. It is important to refer that all ancient traditions and all religions refer to the existence of two things that are contradictory and completely different—heaven and hell.

Paradise is a place where the person whose life has expired in this world (and died) lives in comfort and peace, and he also enjoys all forms of luxury that he desires for himself, unlike hell, which is a place where man tastes the most severe torment and is punished for his bad intentions and all his evil deeds.

Thus, in the other world, there are two different life forms.

One is torment, punishment and misery (hell) and the other contains comfort, peace, happiness and the eternal bliss (paradise).

I know that you, dear reader, would now like to wonder how to avoid hell and enter to paradise.

The condition, dear reader, is simple. If you want to enter paradise and avoid hell, then you, dear reader, must be a good person and positively influential in your society and your surroundings in addition to your sincere belief to God because sincere belief in God is what inspires a person to be a good and positive person in his society and also motivates him to avoid negative actions and words.

So, whatever your financial or social condition, it is important for you, dear reader, not to lose sight of the fact that you will die one day and move to the other world.

Sooner or later, you will die, dear reader, and you will move to the world of spirits where neither money nor power nor a certain authority will benefit you. What will benefit would be your good actions and your good intentions.

So I hope, dear reader, that you do not lose sight of the fact that you will die one day and that you prepare well for that day by being a positive and good person in your society and also make sure that your good deeds are more than your bad deeds because that is what will empower you after God's mercy (and His forgiveness) to enter the paradise and to live in eternal peace.

Every material thing will one day perish, including the human body, so there will be nothing left but yourself, your soul and your (spiritual) heart, which are determined by your actions and intentions (good or bad).

So, dear reader, be careful that your heart is full of moral and noble values and also that your positive influence is stronger than your negative influence in this life.

Death is a fact that each one of us will face when his time comes.

And nobody of us can predict the day of his death.

Even if a person rides in a safe car equipped with all passenger protection devices, and also wears a seatbelt, he can die in a traffic accident (and this has happened in many cases).

Even if a person is also riding on a plane equipped with the latest safety systems, it is possible for him to suffer a fatal accident, such as that plane falling and crashing somewhere.

This has happened in many fatal accidents in which hundreds of people have lost their lives (and I am not inviting you, dear reader, to be pessimistic, or even to a pathological and permanent fear of death, or not to take precaution and pay attention to your safety while you are driving or riding a car of somebody).

No, pessimism is not a good thing, and the pathological and permanent fear of death will also turn your life into continuous torment.

And lack of precaution while driving a car may also cause you to die or expose you to a serious traffic accident that may destroy your life and make you live with a permanent disability.

But all I wanted to assure you, dear reader, is that it is impossible for you to know when you will die because you may die at any time (even if you are on the safest means of transport).

In order for you to understand my meaning well, dear reader, I will tell you the story of the sinking of the Titanic—

that gigantic ship that reaches a height of about 175 feet (54 metres) above sea level, and which most pessimists did not expect to sink on its first voyage.

That story began, dear reader, when the Irish ship designer, Thomas Andrews, decided to design a ship so huge that it would be impossible for it to sink into the sea.

Thus, this ship was designed in a legendary way, as it contained many shock absorbers at the bottom of its hull so that these shocks would work to ensure that water does not enter the inside of that ship in the event of a collision (with something).

This design was implemented after only three years.

Thus, the construction of the Titanic was completed in the year 1912.

That achievement was great in every sense of the word, as this ship is still into today considered as the largest ship ever built in human history.

Vanity dominated both William Perry and Thomas Andrews, who engineered and built the ship to the extent that Andrews said (and frankly) as an answer to a journalist's question (in one of his press interviews) about the degree of safety that this ship provides to its passengers that even God could not drown it.

But the exact opposite is what happened on 10th April (year 1912) after the Titanic took off on its first voyage. After the Titanic left the port of London (heading to New York), the ship observer was surprised when he noticed an iceberg a few miles from the Titanic so that it was impossible to avoid the ship's collision with that iceberg.

This happened on the fourth day of the trip (at exactly 11 o'clock at night) when the Titanic collided with that iceberg in a tragic accident that killed 1,517 people (after the ship's captain, Captain Edward Smith, and his crew failed to avoid that collision).

So the Titanic sank on its first voyage—in a terrible and painful accident that claimed the lives of 1,517 people on that ship. Most of them were nobles (and from the bourgeois class in Europe).

It was a painful accident in every sense of the word, dear reader.

But the point of my narration to you of the details of that catastrophe (the sinking of the Titanic) is to indicate that a person's date of death is in the hands of God only.

None of us knows whether he will die or live. A person may die while sleeping in his bed, and another person may escape from death in a dangerous accident.

Joe Simpson (for example) miraculously escaped death, and today he enjoys his full health and wellness. He even wrote the book *Touching the Void*, in which he tells the details of the incident that happened to him, and more than a million copies were sold from that book, so he became a millionaire and one of the richest people in his country, unlike the nobles of Europe, the 1,517 people who died in the sinking of the Titanic despite the availability of that ship on the latest navigation technology and the best safety systems (for ships) of its time.

So (dear reader) the nobles died while they were on the Titanic, which was called the ship that could not sink, and Joe Simpson (the English mountaineer and author of *Touching the Void*, one of the best-selling books in the world) survived.

The nobles died—no one expected their death (even the most pessimistic)—and Joe Simpson, who everyone expected his death, survived this fatal accident. He also became a millionaire and author of one of the best-selling books in the world.

So, dear reader, none of us guarantees that he will live even one hour in this life because a person may die at any moment and in any time.

I ask you, dear reader, not to misunderstand what I mean. I am not calling you to be pessimistic or to have a constant and toxic fear of death or even to think excessively about it.

No, the point of these two stories I have told you is to draw your attention, dear reader, to the fact that one day, you will die (and I will die too).

Therefore, you and I should prepare well for that day because after the death of a person, nothing will benefit him except his good deeds and his positive and constructive actions.

After the death of a person, no one will remember him except for his actions, if his actions are positive and constructive actions or they are negative and harmful actions to him and his surroundings.

Therefore, the most important thing in this life, dear reader, is the actions of a person and the impact he has in his life.

So it is important for you, dear reader, to pay attention to your actions and to the impact that you do to others.

Because people will not remember you after your death by the money, power, the influence and material things you possessed during your life (whatever they were).

No, they will only mention one thing, and it is certainly your actions (whether they were good, positive, constructive or otherwise).

This is because your positive and constructive actions make a positive impact on others.

Therefore, when your actions are positive and constructive, your memory will stay beautiful in the eyes of others, and your soul will also remain alive within them.

No one will care about what you were doing for yourself (your material possessions, your social status...). Everyone will only care about the extent of your positive impact (on others) because that is what will remain alive after your death (and after your transition to the other world).

Also, when your good deeds are more than your bad deeds, and your positive influence is stronger than your negative influence, you will further elevate your position in the other world and thus guarantee (after the mercy of God) living in eternal peace and bliss and moving to the most beautiful place of all, which is heaven (and also stay away from hell).

Therefore, I would like through this part to alert you, dear reader, to the fact that you will die one day and that you will move after that to the other world where nothing will benefit you except your good deeds, your good intentions and your positive influence on others.

Do not forget, dear reader, that the day will come when you will move to that world. After all, I will die, and you will die, and everyone will die.

So never forget, dear reader, that in the end, you will die (NB: hope to meet each other in the heaven).

Wisdom
Part Seven

After a person dies, people will only remember him for his good deeds and the positive impact he had on them. So it is important for you, dear reader, to make sure that your positive influence on others (and in this life in general) is stronger than your negative influence.

In order to live happily, dear reader, you should adapt to the reality of death and do not be afraid of it (because death is nothing but a transition to the other world). We will all die one day, and after our death, we will find nothing but our good deeds. So, dear reader, be careful that your good deeds are more than your bad deeds and that your positive influence is also stronger than your negative influence (because that is what will enable you, after the mercy of God, to move and go to the most wonderful place, which is heaven.

Conclusion

As a conclusion of your long and interesting journey through the pages of this book, I would like to assure you, passionate reader, that the chemistry of happiness can only be generated in the depths of your heart.

It is the human spiritual heart that controls the secretion of hormones (dopamine and serotonin) in the brain.

That is, man's reconciliation with himself and his harmony with the spirit of the world in which we live and with the laws of life set by God is what will enable him to live happily and comfortably in his life, and it is what will lead him on the path of growth and prosperity and avoid him the path of misery.

So it is important for you, dear reader, to live in reconciliation with yourself and your being and in complete harmony with the laws of life that God has established in order to enjoy that precious and rare thing called true happiness.

Perhaps you would like to wonder about the nature of these laws that I am telling you about, passionate reader (for I did not mention them to you in the parts of book).

But I have mentioned it to you, dear reader, implicitly (and indirectly) in all parts.

The laws that will help you, dear reader, to live properly and live a life full of happiness and peace are as follows:

True happiness you can achieve when you possess noble principles and morals for which you live in addition to having a message in your life.

Work is an essential thing in the life of every human. When a person works (especially in the work he loves), he leads himself on the path of happiness and prosperity (and success as well).

Positive and constructive success that leads its owner to live happily. The motive behind achieving it is the love of good for others and the sincere desire to positively influence the lives of many people.

Thanks and gratitude increase blessings and bring wealth in all its forms. When a person lives a positive life and is thankful to God for His blessings, he leads his life on the path of wealth and prosperity in all its forms.

Change is one of the immutable laws in this life, so there is no way (for man) to try to escape from it or even avoid it. But when a person adapts to the changes and ups and downs of life, he leads himself on the path of success and prosperity in all its forms, which also entitles him to live in true happiness.

The mind is nothing but a tool given to us by God. It is nothing but a biological organ that helps us think properly. But if a person makes his mind his master and follows everything that his mind dictates to him, then he will lead himself in the path of misery. Even mental and neurological diseases. So, following a person to his heart is what leads him to live in happiness and comfort.

Death is a fact of life, and there is no escape from death. In order to live happily, you must adapt to the fact that you will die one day and also avoid the pathological and permanent fear of it.

So, as a conclusion to all of the above, I hope that you have benefitted well, dear reader, from this book that is in your hands, and that it has created a positive and constructive influence within you that enables you to live in lasting happily.

Dear reader, I have tried to convey to you everything I know with sincerity and honesty so that I can help you as much as possible to obtain that precious thing called true happiness.

So I hope you, dear reader, do not forget me in favour of your prayers. I would also like to extend my thanks and appreciation to my dear mother and father and to everyone who helped me write this book (thank you for everything).

In conclusion, I would like to give you, dear reader, my sincere greetings and wishes for health, happiness, peace, success and prosperity in your practical and 'familial' life.

With all my love and appreciation to you, dear reader, for sacrificing your precious time and effort in order to read this book that is in your hands.

Thank you, dear reader, and I wish you a happy life.

Mohammed Maatallaoui